Ministry of Health - National Centre for HIV/AIDS, Dermatology and STD

World Health Organization Representative Office Cambodia

The Continuum of Care for People Living with HIV/AIDS in Cambodia: Linkages and Strengthening in the Public Health System

CASE STUDY

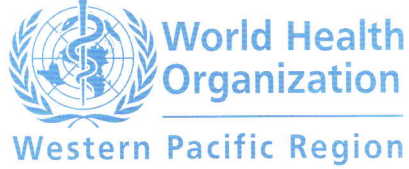

WHO Library Cataloguing in Publication Data

The Continuum of Care for People Living with HIV/AIDS in Cambodia: Linkages and Strengthening in the Public Health System

1. Acquired immunodeficiency syndrome - nursing.
2. HIV infections - nursing.
3. Cambodia

ISBN 92 9061 222 3
(NLM Classification: WY 153.5)

© World Health Organization 2006
All rights reserved.

The designations employed and the presentation of the material in this publication do not imply the expression of any opinion whatsoever on the part of the World Health Organization concerning the legal status of any country, territory, city or area or of its authorities, or concerning the delimitation of its frontiers or boundaries. Dotted lines on maps represent approximate border lines for which there may not yet be full agreement.

The mention of specific companies or of certain manufacturers' products does not imply that they are endorsed or recommended by the World Health Organization in preference to others of a similar nature that are not mentioned. Errors and omissions excepted, the names of proprietary products are distinguished by initial capital letters.

The World Health Organization does not warrant that the information contained in this publication is complete and correct and shall not be liable for any damages incurred as a result of its use.

Publications of the World Health Organization can be obtained from Marketing and Dissemination, World Health Organization, 20 Avenue Appia, 1211 Geneva 27, Switzerland (tel: +41 22 791 2476; fax: +41 22 791 4857; email: bookorders@who.int). Requests for permission to reproduce WHO publications, in part or in whole, or to translate them – whether for sale or for noncommercial distribution – should be addressed to Publications, at the above address (fax: +41 22 791 4806; email: permissions@who.int). For WHO Western Pacific Regional Publications, request for permission to reproduce should be addressed to Publications Office, World Health Organization, Regional Office for the Western Pacific, P.O. Box 2932, 1000, Manila, Philippines, Fax. No. (632) 521-1036, email: publications@wpro.who.int

Contributed by William A. Wells, Ph.D., M.I.A.
Design & Layout: MCD design | design@mcdcambodia.com

Contents

Acronyms   4
Acknowledgements   5
Executive Summary   6
Introduction   8
  I. Background and Rationale for this Case Study   10
  II. Principles underlying the Continuum of Care   11
    II.1. What is the Continuum of Care in Cambodia?   11
    II.2. CoC strategy: A clear plan and linkages   11
      Proposals for further strengthening of CoC linkages   12
    II.3. Cooperative support: Coordinating government,   13
    NGOs, and international partners
      The challenges of NGO coordination in Siem Reap   14
  III. Implementing the Continuum of Care   15
    III.1. How a CoC is started   15
      The first site: the CoC in Moung Russey   15
    III.2. Training to build capacity and allow for expansion   16
      Pediatric Care: An Increasing Priority for the CoC   16
    III.3. Incentives and workload   17
  IV. Linkages to the Community   18
    IV.1. Bringing communities and healthcare providers together   18
    IV.2. The changing face of Home-based care   19
      Changes in HBC   20
      Outreach or transport?   21
    IV.3. PLHA involvement   21
      CPN+ and Self-help groups   22
      How NCHADS coordinates with local partners   22
  V. The Challenges and Potential of Expansion   23
    V.1. Resource constraints: what gives when there is less money?   23
    V.2. Spillovers: Can the CoC cause general health system strengthening?   23
  VI. The Future of the CoC   25
    VI.1. Areas for future expansion   25
      Social sectors and the CoC   25
      Secondary prevention   25
      TB/HIV   25
      PMTCT   25
    VI.2. Financial resources, local leadership, and will   26
Appendix A: Interview subjects   28
References   30
Notes   31

Acronyms

AHC	Angkor Hospital for Children
AIDS	Acquired Immunodeficiency Syndrome
ANC	Ante-Natal Care
ART	Anti-Retroviral Therapy
CBO	Community Based Organization
CENAT	National Center for Tuberculosis and Leprosy Control
CMS	Central Medical Store
CoC	Continuum of Care
CoC-CC	Continuum of Care Coordination Committee
CPN+	Cambodia People Living with HIV/AIDS Network
ESTHER	Ensemble pour une Solidarité Thérapeutique Hospitalière en Réseau
FHI	Family Health International
HBC	Home-Based Care
HIV	Human Immunodeficiency Virus
IPD	Inpatient Department
KHANA	Khmer HIV/AIDS NGO Alliance
MMM	Mondul Mith Chouy Mith (Center for Friends Help Friends)
MSF	Médecins Sans Frontières
NCHADS	National Center for HIV/AIDS, Dermatology and STD
NCMCH	National Center for Maternal and Child Health
NGO	Non-Governmental Organization
OD	Operational District
OI	Opportunistic Infection
OPD	Outpatient Department
OVC	Orphans and Vulnerable Children
PHD	Provincial Health District
PLHA	Person/People Living with HIV/AIDS
PMTCT	Prevention of Mother to Child Transmission
RH	Referral Hospital
STI	Sexually Transmitted Infection
STD	Sexually Transmitted Disease
TB	Tuberculosis
UNAIDS	The Joint United Nations Programme on HIV/AIDS
VCCT	Voluntary, Confidential Counseling and Testing
WHO	World Health Organization

Acknowledgements

Sincere thanks are due to Dr Sor Hong from the Pursat Provincial Health Department for tireless organizing, logistics, and translation. Drs. Mean-Chhi Vun, Massimo Ghidinelli and Nicole Seguy conceived of this project and assisted during the preparation and revision stages. But most of all, thanks are due to the many hard-working CoC staff and PLHA who gave freely of their time and opinions during interviews and focus groups.

Executive Summary

HIV/AIDS is a multifactorial disease requiring life-long treatment. In 2003, Cambodia released its plan to meet this need — the comprehensive Continuum of Care (CoC) — which is an integrated provision of treatment for people living with HIV/AIDS (PLHA). In three short years, Cambodia's National Center for HIV/AIDS and STI (NCHADS) has started and expanded this country-devised and country-led activity. By the end of 2005, it was reaching 20 out of the country's 68 operational districts (ODs), including free antiretroviral treatment (ART) for 11,284 PLHA out of the estimated 19,184 adult Cambodians who currently need it. Additionally 1,071 children are receiving ART.

This case study provides a snapshot of the CoC as it is in the middle of this rapid expansion. It is also an investigation of possible health system strengthening effects achieved by the CoC. In general, the four provinces included in the study had a common understanding of the multiple elements that make up the CoC, despite their varying levels of outside support from non-governmental organizations (NGOs) and donors for implementation.

The main principles underlying the CoC are a strong and consistent plan, local ownership, and links both between different services in the referral hospital and between the community and the referral hospital. These principles have been the foundation for an integrated provision of services including: (1) voluntary confidential counseling and testing (VCCT) services, linking prevention and care; (2) community services (home-based care (HBC) teams and PLHA support groups); (3) health facility-based care (opportunistic infection (OI) treatment and ART for adults and children; tuberculosis (TB)/HIV care and treatment; prevention of mother to child transmission (PMTCT), and laboratory and pharmacy services); and (4) Mondul Mith Chouy Mith (MMM; Center for Friends Help Friends) activities.

> *Establishing the CoC has been a massive undertaking driven by strong leadership, decentralized learning, and participatory and local ownership. It has created an opportunity not only to bring high quality treatment to many PLHA, but also to strengthen the health system and its relationship to the communities that it serves.*

Local, collaborative decision-making is carried out by PLHA, community leaders, NGOs, international partners, and government health staff, who together make up the CoC Coordination Committee (CoC-CC) in each OD. The government health staffs take the lead role. Coordination has depended on the willingness of all of these partners to distribute their efforts rationally, so that existing gaps are filled and all of the CoC Framework can be tackled. The CoC is supported by strong training regimens, including standardized courses in Phnom Penh and exchanges between more and less experienced ODs. The trainings also support laboratory and drug provision systems that are able to answer to rapidly changing needs during the scaling-up phase.

▶

Links to the community have come from three sources. The MMM activities have helped educate PLHA and healthcare providers alike, and create a sense of solidarity and companionship between PLHA. HBC teams identify PLHA or patients in the community, and do drug-adherence monitoring and education of PLHA and community members. Finally, PLHA involvement in the MMM, CoC-CC, and hospital operations help to make them partners rather than passive recipients.

NCHADS focuses first on medical interventions and enlists NGOs to help with some of the links to the community. This makes the formation and maintenance of these community links more of a challenge in ODs where there are few NGOs. These ODs are also more reliant on strong local leaders and clear management practices. If they have these elements, they can maintain the comprehensive CoC despite a generally low level of resources.

There is some evidence for positive spillovers from the CoC to the rest of the health system. The leadership, enthusiasm, and hard work of CoC team members have been noticed by other healthcare workers as an example to follow. But full benefits from improvements in laboratory and pharmacy operations will have to wait, in some locations, for an integration of HIV and non-HIV facilities and personnel. Integration and spillovers will increase in the future if funding mechanisms acknowledge that effective HIV/AIDS treatment can happen only in the context of a strong health system. This acknowledgement should lead to a broad interpretation of how HIV funding can and should be spent.

Introduction

Cambodia's healthcare manpower and infrastructure were decimated in 16 years of war and neglect — from the 1975 entry of the Khmer Rouge into Phnom Penh until the 1991 signing of the Paris Peace Accords. 1991 was also the year that the country's first case of HIV infection was detected. HIV prevalence in adults rose quickly to 3.0% in 1997, but declined in response to a successful 100% condom campaign, targeted outreach to commercial sex workers and their clients, and high AIDS-related mortality. Based on 2003 figures, Cambodia has HIV prevalence among adults of 1.9%, reflecting 123,100 adults with HIV and 19,184 estimated to have AIDS.

With HIV prevention gaining traction, and prices of antiretroviral drugs falling, the next logical step was HIV/AIDS treatment. Anti-retroviral treatment (ART) was introduced in 2001, but was restricted to a few large hospitals in major urban centers, which established vertical cohorts of patients with limited linkages to communities.

To create a more comprehensive and sustainable system, Cambodia's remarkable response was the Continuum of Care (CoC), whose expansion is documented here. The CoC was designed and driven by a highly motivated team from Cambodia's National Center for HIV/AIDS and STI (NCHADS) led by its director Dr. Mean-Chhi Vun. For the first time it united the efforts of clinicians and people living with HIV/AIDS (PLHA), resulting in district-based services that emphasized team work, community linkages, and a public health approach.

The CoC Operational Framework, outlining a national plan for free HIV/AIDS treatment and care, was published by NCHADS in April 2003.[1] This was at a time when the challenges in Cambodia were legion.[2] Internationally, there was "limited evidence of the feasibility and effectiveness of [anti-retroviral treatment in resource-limited settings] outside of [a] few small studies."[3] Brazil had been a notable success,[4] but this was based on a budget and human-resource base that was far above what was available in Cambodia.

Nevertheless, by the end of 2005, a total of 20 operational districts (ODs) in Cambodia were implementing all or part of the CoC, with 15 more to be added during 2006. By the end of 2005, the CoC included ART for 12,355 PLHA (including 1071 children), and 2005 saw a total of 13,775 new patients starting on therapy for opportunistic infections (OIs). By 2010, 40 out of Cambodia's 68 ODs should be operating the CoC service-delivery model.

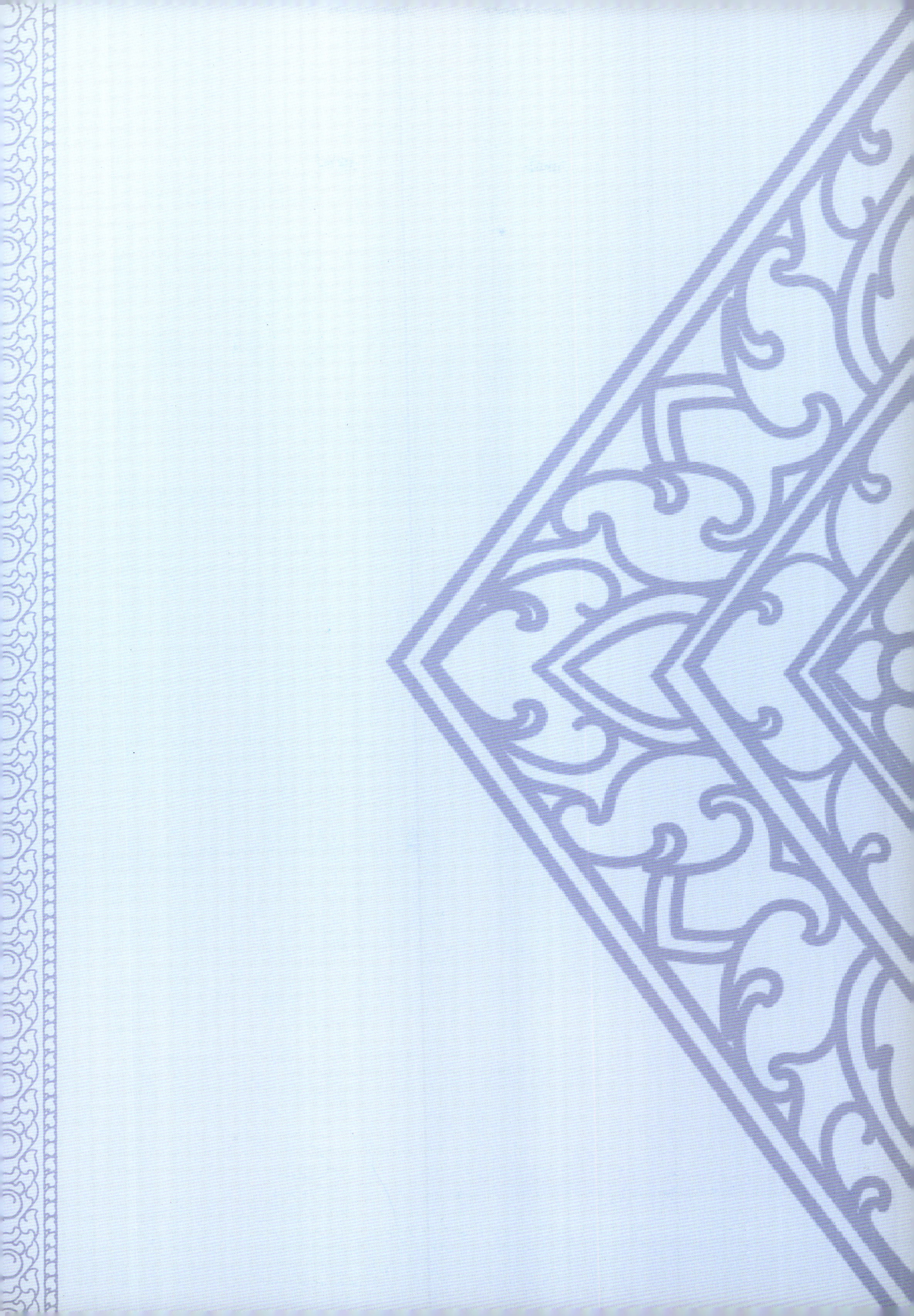

I. Background and Rationale for this Case Study

Several publications have documented CoC implementation experiences in Cambodia. A study in 2004 described the process in Moung Russey OD (Battambang Province), the first OD to implement the CoC.[5] Proceedings of an inter-country CoC workshop, based in Battambang Province, were published in 2005.[6] And Family Health International (FHI) has recently published a DVD ("5 Lives") describing the CoC implementation in Moung Russey.

The current case study aims to provide a snapshot of the CoC as it is in the midst of expanding from a single OD to a country-wide exercise in strengthening the healthcare system. There is considerable interest in the potential for HIV/AIDS activities to contribute to health system strengthening, and in determining how system-weakening effects can be avoided.[7]

This case study focuses on organizational rather than technical issues and does not attempt to evaluate the standard of care. For this reason, sections below are grouped around themes of management and strategy rather than treatment modality. (For a more extensive discussion of each medical element of the CoC, see the 2004 "Cambodia Cares" study.[5]) A section on overarching principles is followed by a discussion of implementation strategies, including community linkages. Challenges of expanding into a resource-poor OD are discussed before considering possible system-strengthening effects and future trends.

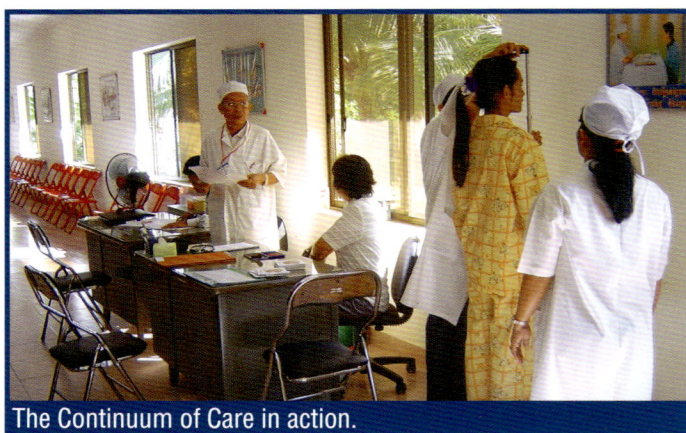
The Continuum of Care in action.

Only limited time was available for data collection, so not all points below were confirmed by more than one source, and only 4 ODs were visited. Finally, although Cambodia's approach has included integration of care and prevention efforts, prevention efforts were not investigated and are not described in detail in this document.

Information was collected via key informant interviews in Phnom Penh, and key informant and provider interviews and PLHA focus groups at the 4 provincial sites. The 4 ODs outside of Phnom Penh that were visited were:

◆ Moung Russey, where the CoC was established first and with considerable support from FHI;
◆ Siem Reap, where establishment of the CoC was preceded by OI treatment and ART activities by other, non-governmental actors;
◆ Svay Rieng, where the CoC was established in a provincial capital with limited outside help;
◆ Neak Loeung, where the CoC was established far from Prey Veng, the provincial capital, and with limited outside help.

Based on a rapid assessment, the essential elements of the CoC appear to have been consistently applied in the ODs under study. Below are detailed the most important elements of the CoC as it is applied in the field, and some examples of how it is adapting to new circumstances as they are encountered.

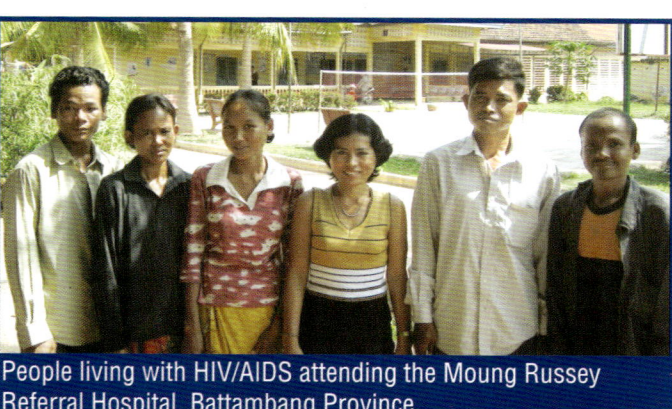
People living with HIV/AIDS attending the Moung Russey Referral Hospital, Battambang Province.

Continuum of Care for People Living with HIV/AIDS in Cambodia

II. Principles underlying the Continuum of Care

II.1. What is the Continuum of Care in Cambodia?

The portrayal of ART as an easy and quick fix for HIV/AIDS is misleading. Any successful HIV/AIDS care model requires multiple elements,[8,9] and a strong health system to implement those elements. The Cambodian CoC is an extraordinary response to an extraordinary public health challenge.

A country like Cambodia faces numerous challenges when starting a service-delivery model for HIV/AIDS care. NCHADS, the relevant central authority in Cambodia, is part of an HIV/AIDS field that is crowded with many players who have many divergent priorities.[10] In hospitals, clinicians with limited training face complications including drug side-effects, drug resistance, and the wide array of OIs with which a PLHA may first present. Community complications include the need to identify patients and to promote education that ensures regular hospital visits, drug adherence, and safe sex even when the PLHA is feeling better.

The key feature of the CoC in Cambodia is that it is built around linkages. These linkages are needed because of the nature of AIDS itself — it is a chronic disease, and its management requires services that are provided by a wide array of health workers. The CoC thus links the workers in these different areas of the hospital, and links the hospital to the community so that patients can be identified and followed over time.

Both the linkages within the hospital and from hospital to community were weak before the CoC was established. The majority of community members seeking care looked first to unlicensed private providers or pharmacies rather than health centers and referral hospitals. And the health system was, as in many resource-constrained settings, dominated by vertical services that communicated little with each other.

Multiple elements of the CoC have helped link the community to the health care system, including home-based care (HBC),[11] the CoC Coordination Committee (CoC-CC), and the Mondul Mith Chouy Mith (MMM; Center for Friends Help Friends) activities of PLHA and community and medical leaders. These events and organizations bring in non-governmental organizations (NGOs), PLHA, and community and religious leaders as full actors in the treatment strategy. Further details on each of these elements appear below.

Within each referral hospital, linkages between services were made a necessity by the multi-factorial nature of AIDS itself. PLHA require services from units devoted to voluntary confidential counseling and testing (VCCT),[12] prevention of mother to child transmission (PMTCT), treatment of tuberculosis (TB), sexually transmitted infections (STIs), and OIs, provision of ART, laboratory testing, imaging, and pharmacy. The presence of a large group of individuals requiring these multiple services, and the existence of the CoC Framework, have provided the catalyst for new linkages.

II.2. CoC strategy: A clear plan and linkages

"This is a Cambodian program. We designed the program, so we have the vision."
Dr. Mean Chhi Vun, Director, NCHADS.

The essential starting point for the CoC was a well-defined plan. Critically, this plan was devised by Cambodians for Cambodians, with inputs from partners contributing as needed. The plan had to be clear not only to those at the center who devised it, but to three other critical groups: international partners; provincial and district implementing officials; and local communities. The participation of all three of these groups was needed to make the CoC work, and the starting point for that participation was a plan that was perceived consistently throughout the country.

This consistency is defined in part through standardized forms and guidelines that are devised centrally. But to translate the CoC into practice, local ownership is crucial. The naming is always consistent – with the CoC now being identified as 'good' the district officials are keen to publicize that they have adopted 'CoC'. But it is the sharing of experiences across provinces that has continually reminded district health officials that a comprehensive CoC includes a multitude of elements.

II. Principles underlying the Continuum of Care

Once the plan is in place, the linkages between all of the CoC services are provided via standardized mechanisms and referral forms and, at some sites, facilitated by PLHA volunteers who guide other PLHA from one area of the referral hospital to another. Cooperation was initiated centrally, with NCHADS identifying common areas of work between its AIDS Care Unit and:

♦ the National Center for Tuberculosis and Leprosy Control (CENAT);
♦ the STI unit of NCHADS;
♦ the National Centre for Maternal and Child Health (NCMCH) unit involved in PMTCT;
♦ the National Mental Health Program for mental health.

Originally, stand-alone operation was common even for those services, such as VCCT and PMTCT, that have always had a clear thematic link to HIV prevention and care. These services have now been drawn into the CoC system. Linkages that currently exist include:

♦ VCCT to OI/ART.
This is for same-day referral.
♦ ante-natal care (ANC)/PMTCT to OI/ART.
This is for same-day referral.
♦ HBC teams to referral hospital.
HBC teams refer suspected cases to VCCT, and serious cases to the inpatient department (IPD). Hospital staffs notify HBC teams of those who have missed appointments, so that the teams can do follow-up. Finally, HBC team members participate on the ART selection committee, as they know the home situation well, and can work with the committee to find adherence solutions. This also makes them aware of which PLHA are beginning ART.
♦ OI/ART to PLHA support groups.
Communication between these groups is mediated by the NGO Cambodia People Living with HIV/AIDS Network (CPN+), which gives OI/ART information to the support groups, convenes monthly meetings of their leaders, and communicates any conclusions of these meetings to the CoC-CC and OI/ART team.
♦ VCCT and OI/ART to TB.
There is TB screening of all suspected cases of TB among HIV-infected people, and of all consenting TB patients for HIV.
♦ VCCT and PMTCT to STI, and vice versa.

These linkages are not just functional but help the services to strengthen each other. Two of the visited sites have seen a doubling of VCCT clients over the 1-2 years during which ART was introduced. This may be a common finding throughout the country.

Proposals for further strengthening of CoC linkages

Interviewees suggested several approaches to ensure that CoC linkages are further strengthened. One key area is to maintain and improve the function of the CoC-CC and OI/ART team in defining exactly who is responsible for each link in the procedural chain. With general lab diagnostic tests, for example, NGO staff stressed that a procedure is needed to ensure that test requests and results are processed promptly, and that there are mechanisms to detect any delays. Any successful management strategies of this kind should then be spread to the referral hospital's other departments (see "Spillovers" section, below). OI/ART team leaders at several sites suggested that routine case conferences can act as a check to see whether these chains of operation are working successfully. These management initiatives can be introduced by local staff; the best way to prompt this may be exchange visits where staff can see different practices in other settings.

The CoC presumes that most people will enter the system via VCCT and its link to the OI/ART team, and indeed this is true for many PLHA. Yet many others present only when they are already very sick, and do so first at the OPD.

This raises two issues. First, in the OPD the training on common OI symptoms is sometimes lacking due to the limited size of the OI/ART team (see below). This challenge can be addressed without a full-scale training of all hospital staff in Phnom Penh. Svay Rieng staff suggested that the OI/ART team conduct a short course to inform other referral hospital staff about basic HIV/AIDS symptoms and care, and the referral mechanisms available within the hospital.

Second, UNICEF staff suggested that the number of people going to VCCT might be raised by using new types of promotional materials.

II. Principles underlying the Continuum of Care

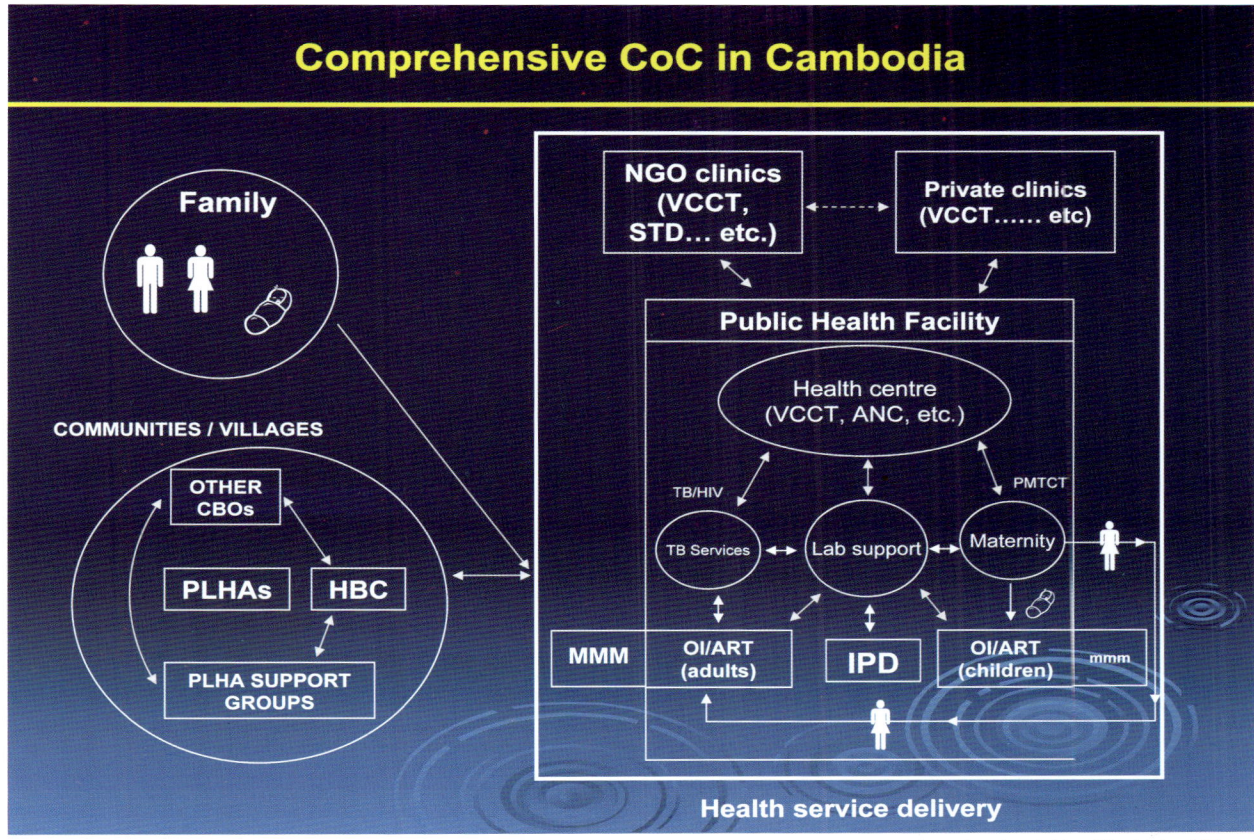

*MMM: Mondul Mith Chouy Mith (Center for Friends Help Friends) for adults. *mmm: Mondul Mith Chouy Mith (Center for Friends He p Friends) for children.

Education campaigns could be directed not just at getting people to use VCCT but at promoting the care available, the benefits and challenges of ART, the benefits of getting care early, and how to access this care.

II.3. Cooperative support: Coordinating government, NGOs, and international partners

A final principle is coordination. In a service-delivery model as large as the CoC, coordination of funding and technical support is critical. Two strategies at the central level have made this work:

♦ inclusion of all partners in the planning phase; but
♦ clear ownership of the CoC by the Royal Government of Cambodia (RGC) and NCHADS.

The result of these strategies has been clarity: one plan that is followed by all partners; and cooperation of all partners with NCHADS to fill gaps and avoid overlap. The leadership from NCHADS has been essential in coordinating partners to support a rapid scale-up.

International partners must continue to adhere to a single definition of the CoC. It is possible that individual provinces will periodically lose support from one partner and gain it from another. But the real confusion arises, at all levels of the health system, if the new partner decides to support a different set of interventions or incentives. Compliance with the provisions of the CoC framework ensures consistency and makes for stronger partnerships.

The same inclusive strategy that is used centrally works also at the provincial level with the CoC-CC, which draws on healthcare staff from multiple departments. The CoC-CC involves important community and healthcare leaders, so doctors on the OI/ART team have a strong incentive to

II. Principles underlying the Continuum of Care

perform. The involvement of PLHA, monks, and community leaders also keeps the community and healthcare workers informed about each other's concerns. NGOs can also raise issues, or invite the OD to help in supervision.

NGOs have several potential roles. For HBC, NGOs provide the connection to the community. For OI/ART, NGOs can assist with technical support.

The challenges of NGO coordination in Siem Reap

Coordination of multiple actors is achieved at the CoC-CC. This job is particularly challenging when NGOs have established services before any government services exist. Siem Reap is a prime example of these complications. As a large provincial center and tourist destination, it has attracted a variety of non-government actors. These actors are providing valuable and often high quality services, but they make navigating the healthcare system more complicated for both government administrators and patients. The interactions of these actors with the government system range from extensive to almost zero.

For example, within Siem Reap Referral Hospital, Médecins Sans Frontières (MSF) has been supplying OI treatment since 2002 and ART since 2003, with many patients traveling from far away. In the same building, across a narrow corridor from MSF, are OD staff supported by the French program ESTHER (Ensemble pour une Solidarité Thérapeutique Hospitalière en Réseau, which twins North and South hospitals to support ART provision). These OD staff started OI/ART services in early 2003, just before CoC protocols were released, and now provide CoC services. At a more distant site within Siem Reap town, the NGO-funded Angkor Hospital for Children (AHC) has been providing pediatric ART since 2003.

Organizational principles for the institutions vary. ESTHER-supported OD staff are recruited locally, get close to the standard government salaries, and see patients only in the morning. MSF staff, however, are drawn from all over the country, paid an undisclosed salary, and see patients both morning and afternoon. Relations between the two groups improved when they participated in trainings together, but in general the differing conditions may limit exchange and learning opportunities.

The 2003 issuance of the CoC Framework introduced some new concepts and some old concepts with altered procedures. For example, the clinician meetings and PLHA groups run by MSF have evolved into the more inclusive CoC-CC and MMM formats. The enthusiasm of non-government actors for these new procedures has been variable. The MMM adaptation, for example, has taken some time, and only recently has it included PLHA from all treatment centers and taken on some of the key features of other MMMs. Healthcare workers at non-government sites are still confused, however, about whether this is "like any other meeting, with the same faces." It is also taking time to rationalize outside funding (such as ESTHER funding to the entire referral hospital) with the NCHADS incentives to the OI/ART team. Any policy change by one funding source has a ripple effect with the other actors, and makes it more challenging for central planners to determine what is happening at the provincial level.

Successful coordination depends on individual personalities — both institutional and personal. The Siem Reap experience suggests that flexibility is needed on both sides. Activities that are given different names by government and NGO staff may turn out to be very similar in intent if not in details, allowing for integration. Government may have to adapt to a changed environment created by the earlier NGO activities, which will inevitably establish a particular set of patient expectations. In turn, NGOs must take into account the need for government staff to use as standardized an approach as possible. With this dialogue in place, the government and NGO staff can learn from each other's experiences.

III. Implementing the Continuum of Care

III.1. How a CoC is started

The CoC is based at the OD level. This stands between the health center, which is close to client populations but has a staff with limited training, and the provincial hospital, which has high technical capacity but is far from many clients. In each OD, a single referral hospital is the site for all clinical treatment and the MMM. The provincial health department (PHD) provides overall technical support, while delegating responsibilities for ongoing operations to OD officials.

CoC implementation begins with a baseline assessment of available resources (existing HBC teams, hospital equipment, human resources, clinical training, and partners). Next comes a sensitization workshop with all partners to generate a single definition of what constitutes a CoC. Roles and positions are defined, leading to a CoC orientation workshop. The CoC-CC is formed and meets to identify teams that implement first MMM activities, then treatment of OIs, and finally ART. PMTCT and TB/HIV strategies are added as resources become available.

The major inputs that NCHADS provides locally include forms and guidelines that outline standard treatment and management protocols, a variety of training courses for each member of a 7-9–person OI/ART team, and performance-based salary incentives of US$60/month to each member of this team.

The first site: the CoC in Moung Russey

Moung Russey OD was the first site to implement the CoC, with the close collaboration and assistance of different partners, including FHI. This demonstration site had to be a success, but it had to be a Cambodian success. Only if the project was perceived as a locally owned achievement, and not an FHI achievement, would the other ODs feel that this was attainable for them too.

Therefore the planning and coordination mechanism — the CoC-CC — included a wide array of local leaders, PHD and OD officials, and PLHA. The CoC-CC helped translate the plan identified by the CoC Framework into a list of actions. NGOs and international partners were then asked to modify their own goals so that they could fill identified gaps in the CoC plan. The local officials understood the CoC from the beginning, because they were running it from the beginning. Training followed a cascade model from the PHD to OD to community level. The initial trainings rewarded participants with knowledge and incentives, and formed a basis for their feeling of ownership.

The first MMM day at Moung Russey was an important moment. For the first time, PLHA had a forum in which they could criticize the care they received from hospital staff, and they did so. The leadership at the referral hospital committed to starting a new attitude from that day onwards, and the PLHA were encouraged by these efforts to include them in the dialogue.

The expansion of the CoC beyond Moung Russey is bringing multiple benefits. As more sites provide OI/ART, more patients are treated. The new sites are also taking the pressure off the older sites, where waiting times for ART are shortening or disappearing. The remaining PLHA at the older CoC sites live on average closer to the referral hospital, resulting in reduced transportation costs and increased treatment adherence.

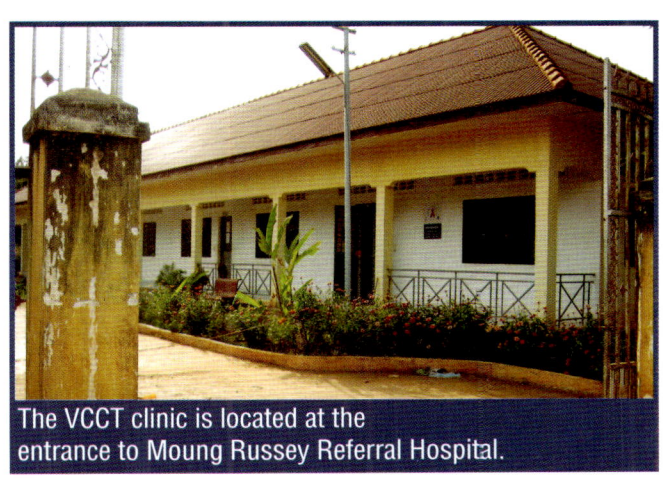

The VCCT clinic is located at the entrance to Moung Russey Referral Hospital.

III. Implementing the Continuum of Care

III.2. Training to build capacity and allow for expansion

"We are training and doing at the same time."
Lyma Virakrith, Deputy of Referral Hospital and OI/ART Team Leader, Neak Loeung.

The OI/ART team is usually a group of 7-9 individuals in a variety of positions, such as 2-3 clinicians, 2-3 counselors, 1 pharmacist, 1 X-ray technician, and 1 lab staff. Although the general roles are described by NCHADS, the means by which they are selected is not specified. This allows flexibility, but can result in a single individual choosing team members who are not the most relevant or qualified.

The team may be expanded based on either additional NGO support or increased case-loads. To avoid the OI/ART team becoming an exclusive club (in terms of both knowledge and salary), mechanisms to spread the knowledge gained by this team are also needed.

CoC training is a combination of standard courses based in Phnom Penh and inter-province exchanges. In Neak Loeung, for example, training for clinicians includes:

♦ the standard initial NCHADS clinical training of 11 weeks spread over 5 months in Phnom Penh;
♦ a specific phone contact in Phnom Penh for OI/ART queries;
♦ follow-up from Prey Veng PHD or NCHADS every week or 2 weeks to check for questions arising;
♦ exchange with Svay Rieng OI/ART team to train on specimen collection for CD4 counts.

Establishing the initial training course has been a major investment and has turned into a major asset for the country. The curriculum is based on alternating classroom and field practice, and covers proficiency in OI prophylaxis, diagnosis and treatment of HIV-related disease, and the use of antiretroviral drugs. Approximately 100 Cambodian medical doctors have attended the 3 training courses given so far; a fourth is now underway.

Updated training and exchanges are needed on an ongoing basis as clinicians gradually encounter the wide range of HIV management challenges. With ART, there is a progression of issues: first with initial ART side-effects; then with longer term side-effects (e.g., lipoatrophy); and finally with treatment failure (viral resistance). Ongoing training and monitoring by physicians from Phnom Penh is limited by time and money. Instead, much of the feedback must come via exchange visits within and between provinces. These have already proven extremely useful. The exchanges result not only in training of the visitors but in increased pride and ownership of the CoC by those hosting the trainees. Sites that today are receiving training by other provinces will, in the future, be giving training to the newest CoC sites. This builds further confidence and ownership at the teaching sites. Institution of regional clinician networks may also help increase the communication between different sites.

Exchanges are also effective for changing norms. NGO staff indicated that, in some locations, poor clinical practices may become accepted, and thus never be questioned by the workers at that location. Exchange of clinicians between different sites should help correct such problems. Thus, although the availability of phone support is a good first step, the ongoing exchanges of clinicians will be vital in continuing the spread of good clinical practice.

Finally, clinician confidence increases as patient intakes improve. Some of the first PLHA to be treated in a given location were also the sickest (with serious OIs and negligible CD4 counts), and thus had poor treatment outcomes. Deaths at a CoC site that had just introduced OI/ART were discouraging to both clinicians and PLHA. But with the increase in numbers of PLHA

Pediatric Care: An Increasing Priority for the CoC

HIV in Cambodia has swept through the sex workers, to the men who used them, to their wives, and now to their children. At Neak Loeung referral hospital, 5 randomly selected individuals from the OI/ART clinic were asked to join a focus group discussion. In 3 of the 5 cases it was the accompanying children who were getting treatment.

All of the children in these three families were brought to Neak Loeung for HIV testing by HBC teams. This emphasizes the importance of identification of PLHA by HBC teams, which were also cited for their ability to reduce stigma in local communities. The participants had heard of plans for a pediatric MMM at Neak Loeung because the regular MMM was getting so noisy with all the children.

A framework for pediatric OI/ART coverage has been published by NCHADS and a training curriculum will be forthcoming. Training that was until recently only done in Thailand will now be done in Phnom Penh, and those newly trained individuals will be added to the OI/ART team at the OD level.

III. Implementing the Continuum of Care

attending OI/ART, presentations may occur at earlier stages of HIV disease and treatment outcomes are likely to improve.

III.3. Incentives and workload

On top of the training, NCHADS provides performance-based salary incentives of US$60/month to each member of the OI/ART team. The size and composition of this team reflects a realistic assessment of the manpower needed to carry out care and treatment at facility level. By spreading the incentives to individuals in different specialties, the CoC helps to integrate the staff's efforts. But at the same time the CoC cannot be expected to fund the entire hospital workforce. Where this line is drawn is by necessity somewhat arbitrary.

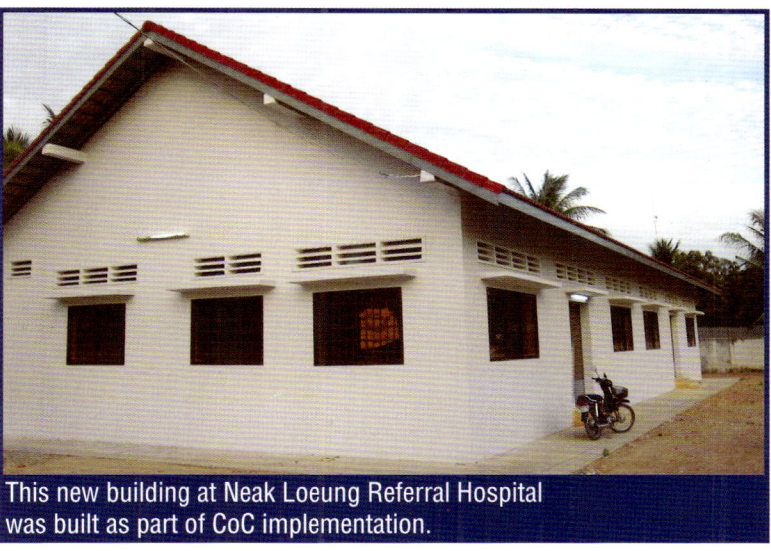

This new building at Neak Loeung Referral Hospital was built as part of CoC implementation.

Civil service workers in Cambodia, including doctors, receive very low pay; this inevitably drives workers into private work. Incentives for the OI/ART doctors are clearly needed to compensate them for the extra hours of work that they spend at the referral hospital specifically working as part of the OI/ART team – otherwise they would be spending this time earning far more money seeing private patients. These doctors accept the burden of the extra work and the bonus of the extra money as a single package. Thus the money is serving the appropriate function of bringing both doctors and patients into the hospital system.

Although there were some mild feelings of jealousy from other doctors, in general the non-OI/ART doctors recognized that the OI/ART team spent more time working and needed to be compensated for this.

The incentives for the non-physician members of the OI/ART team are slightly more troublesome. In many cases these staff members share work spaces and work duties with colleagues who are not part of the OI/ART team. Those who are not on the OI/ART teams miss out in two ways: they do not get the OI/ART incentive; and they do not get the usual share of fees when PLHA are treated, as PLHA get free treatment. Depending on individual personalities, this can lead to bad feelings and inefficient work practices, for example if the staff who are not on the OI/ART team refuse to do any PLHA-related work. In the end a full integration of these staff will rely on equalizing salaries, but for now the incentives are allowing the OI/ART team to get their job done.

Problems with incentives may be lessened in referral hospitals with Health Equity Funds (HEFs). The HEFs pay treatment fees for poorer patients, and in several locations have significantly increased hospital income and salaries by attracting more patients.

IV. Linkages to the Community

IV.1. Bringing communities and healthcare providers together: the MMM experience

A healthcare system cannot operate in isolation from its community. Even the most perfectly engineered HIV care unit will be short of patients if stigma against PLHA is high in the community (and in the hospital), or if the community is unaware of what the hospital has to offer. Links from the healthcare system to the community are central to the CoC. Whereas other service-delivery models may introduce community links in isolated sites, the CoC is unusual in that it has made community links a central theme throughout the entire country.

Going into the first CoC implementation efforts, Cambodia had the advantage that HBC teams were established in many communities, so PLHA were not completely isolated. But the Mondul Mith Chouy Mith (MMM; Center for Friends Help Friends) half-day meetings and activities have been crucial in further strengthening the link between PLHA and the hospital. Before these activities, healthcare providers had little knowledge of the PLHA's non-clinical troubles: their daily struggles and their gaps in medical understanding.

MMM initially used a simple formula to attract people – free food – but the activities became so valuable in forming a community of PLHA that many PLHA now sacrifice a full day and considerable sums of money for travel to make it to each MMM. All participants sit on the floor so that there is no hierarchy, and those who have come from far away are prioritized to have their medical check-ups.

MMM has helped eliminate stigma in the referral hospital. PLHA now carry their special treatment booklets openly, register their names for MMM willingly, and consent to interviews and pictures for publication without a second thought. In more isolated communities, however, stigma remains an issue. Some villagers refuse to buy food from suspected PLHA, or prohibit their children from playing with those of a PLHA. Many PLHA are not open in the community and thus may avoid attending MMM or risk adherence failure because they won't take ART in front of others. But involvement of community leaders in MMM and visits of HBC teams are gradually breaking down this stigma so that AIDS is seen as just another chronic disease.

Stigma is still one of the factors limiting MMM attendance. The Siem Reap MMM, for example, attracts 80-100 PLHA, out of the 2400 PLHA

> ### MMM in Pursat
>
> For the MMM in Pursat, the room is packed, the crowd is noisy, and the sense of community is so thick it can almost be touched. Any newcomer is met by clapping. It is at first disorganized, but amongst laughter and shouts it quickly coalesces into a special rhythm – the MMM clap.
>
> The more formal agenda is delivered in short segments. Healthcare providers, PLHA volunteers, and community leaders talk about adherence to drug regimens, the need to prevent transmission to others even when the drugs make you feel healthy, and the need to attend check-ups regularly. Small groups confer about the problem for the day – transport to the hospital, or side-effect management – and come up with lists of questions and suggestions for the hospital staff. Silence finally falls when a monk leads the group in meditation; he encourages the group to find an inner peace that can be used in times of need.
>
> There is a snack break and a lunch break, and money at the end for transport. Throughout, there is exchange of information and companionship. The participants come away with a strong feeling that the hospital staff do not resent the workload from the CoC, but instead want these people here so that they can work with them, in partnership.

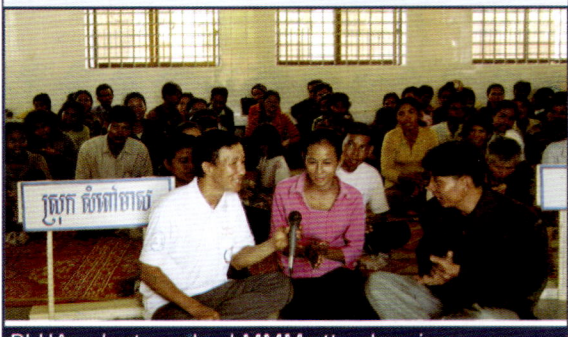

PLHA volunteers lead MMM attendees in song.

IV. Linkages to the Community

treated by MSF Belgium and 880 treated by ESTHER. Transport is another limitation. In many sites the budget allows only 100 PLHA to receive the $1-2 transport allowance for each MMM, although there may be 600 or more PLHA covered by that referral hospital. With more NGOs supporting transport, Battambang town attracts over 300 PLHA to its MMM. But other sites have had to rotate the allowance, with PLHA attending the MMM every few months rather than every month.

Finally, MMM attendance is also limited by the physical space available. Thus a given site may have 2 or more MMMs each month to accommodate all PLHA at least once. These activities may be held at different sites to bring them closer to different groups of PLHA, thus reducing travel costs.

IV.2. The changing face of Home-based care

There are two things that CoC participants – from OD directors to clinicians to PLHA community activists – all agree upon: the importance of HBC; and the need for its further expansion. The nature of HBC is also being re-examined. NCHADS issues guidelines to help the many local NGOs that provide HBC. But with the huge number of these organizations, HBC is one of the less standardized parts of the CoC.

HBC was an initial response to the HIV/AIDS epidemic. It was implemented before OI treatment and ART were available at the referral hospitals, and used teams to provide palliative care in the home. A typical rural HBC team includes 1 part-time health center staff, 2 NGO staff, 1 PLHA, and 1 volunteer per village visited.

When OI/ART treatment started, the focal point for treatment shifted to the referral hospital. This has changed the rationale for HBC to a new but even more vital arena. HBC provides the link between patients in the community and clinicians in the referral hospital – clinicians who are trying to provide a complex, long-term regimen of treatment to patients who start out with limited knowledge of HIV/AIDS. HBC teams help identify new patients in the community, refer them to the hospital, and then track their health status and treatment adherence.

There are many desirable services provided by a subset of HBC teams, including income-generation activities, establishment of PLHA self-help groups, and provision of socio-economic support (shelter, food, and clothes) and psycho-social support. These activities tend to vary depending on the NGO involved, and are difficult to standardize.

But there are three core HBC activities that are absolutely required for the CoC to work properly: identifying PLHA or potential patients in the community (including TB cases that should be tested for HIV); adherence monitoring; and the consistent dissemination of multiple public health messages.

The HBC team identifies individuals who may have HIV/AIDS based on local knowledge of who has been sick, or whose partner has recently died, and encourages these people to seek treatment. In a country with such low utilization of health facilities, this may be the first time that the individual has had any contact with the referral hospital.

Adherence monitoring is needed because ART is a life-long and complex therapy. Providers of TB treatment responded to similar complexity by using Directly Observed Treatment, Short-course

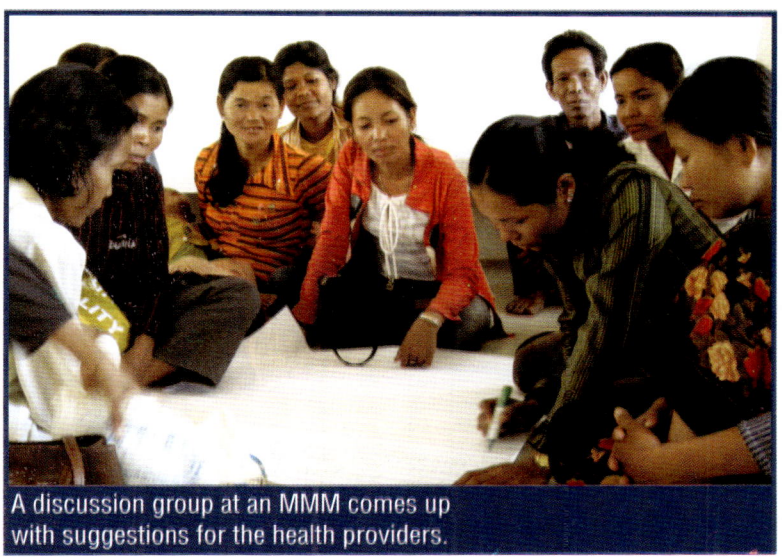

A discussion group at an MMM comes up with suggestions for the health providers.

IV. Linkages to the Community

(DOTS). ART approaches in some countries have used similar methods of direct observation,[13] but many, like Cambodia, use other strategies. The CoC encourages adherence with a combination of:

- requiring PLHA to attend OI/ART clinics for 3 weekly sessions before becoming eligible for ART;
- providing drug counseling and adherence messages during these sessions, and scoring the patient's knowledge;
- home visits by HBC teams;
- delivering adherence reinforcement messages at MMM.

HBC teams provide information to PLHA who are dealing with a prolonged, often challenging course of treatment. If a PLHA misses an appointment, the HBC team is informed by the referral hospital and helps to find the PLHA.

The required public health messages are complex for any community. They include assurances that:

- effective AIDS treatments are available;
- TB, OI and ART medications must be taken regularly even after symptoms improve;
- TB patients and pregnant women should get HIV tests; and
- ART side-effects can be managed and should not prevent a PLHA from getting further treatment.

PLHA who are in areas not covered by HBC either never come to the referral hospital (especially if they are poorer) or come only once they are extremely sick. Because they start ART so late, they may die despite correct treatment. If the ART does make them feel better, they often stop taking the drugs and stop visiting the referral hospital because they presume they are cured. Some areas in Moung Russey have recently lost HBC because of de-funding of a corrupt HBC NGO. OD staff report many subsequent problems with drug adherence in these areas.

Changes in HBC

With CoC expansion, there are three forces encouraging a shift in how HBC is delivered. First is the change in HBC emphasis described above, from palliative care to outreach and identifying PLHA or patients in the community. The second is the pressure for more comprehensive coverage to match the coverage of the CoC, despite a limited budget. Finally, OI/ART teams are turning out a cohort of well-informed, healthy, and community-minded PLHA who are keen to contribute.

PLHA giving HBC: From receiving care to giving care

There are many parallels in the stories of Long Socheat and Prom Chan. Both lost their partners (presumably to AIDS), their livelihoods, and their health. Thankfully both are now on ART, feeling better, and working as volunteers at WOMEN in Ba Phnom, Prey Veng Province, providing home-based care to other PLHA.

Socheat got tested for HIV in Phnom Penh in 1998 just after her husband died. She was sick every day, at one stage being put on oxygen because of her pneumonia. She had already lost all her money paying for the treatment and care for her husband. Meanwhile she lost her job as a restaurant cook when the owner found out she had AIDS. Now, working for WOMEN, she says she has "a very good feeling. I still survive because of their support."

Chan was working in construction before his wife died in 2003; by then he could no longer work because of his own sickness. "I could not even sit; I was always sleeping," he says. After he started ART in May 2005 he felt better and asked to volunteer at WOMEN. He has his own fund-raising plans for the organization so that it can reach even more people in more communities.

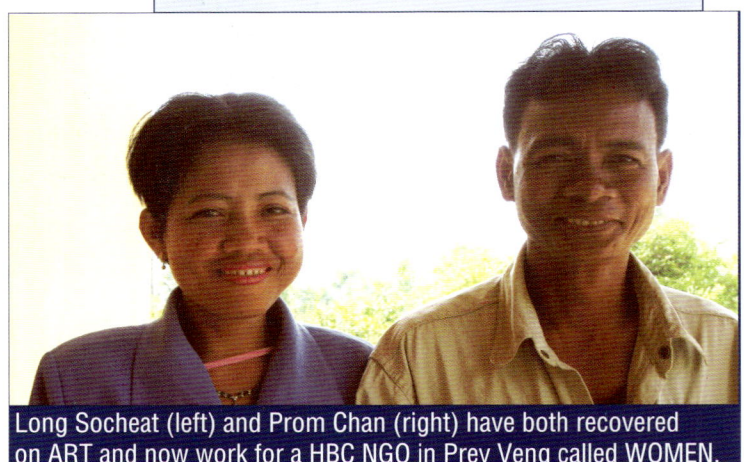

Long Socheat (left) and Prom Chan (right) have both recovered on ART and now work for a HBC NGO in Prey Veng called WOMEN.

IV. Linkages to the Community

These forces have led NCHADS to revise the guidelines for HBC to further emphasize PLHA involvement, including different options for team composition. As some HBC organizations are realizing, PLHA should be used to staff as many of the HBC NGO positions as possible. Many local NGOs that focus on HBC initially used non-PLHA as their core staff – a strategy that made sense when most PLHA were sick most of the time. But PLHA who are getting OI treatment and ART, and who have the required literacy skills, should be able to handle HBC work with only minor reductions in the standard work load. PLHA involvement helps provide jobs and boost self-esteem in this community. HBC staff noted that the PLHA who are currently on HBC teams have proven to be very effective case finders in their communities.

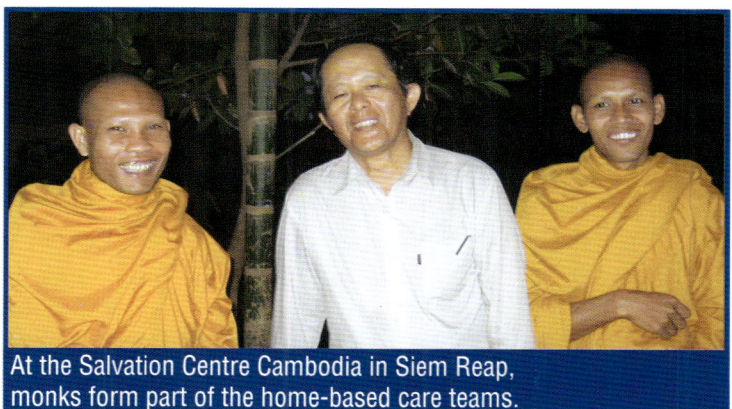

At the Salvation Centre Cambodia in Siem Reap, monks form part of the home-based care teams.

In some ODs there are not enough HBC teams to cover all areas. Under new NCHADS guidelines, these areas may benefit from greater use of 'home-visit' teams consisting only of local PLHA. Training will be needed for such PLHA-only teams, but a base of knowledge exists through the experiences of the PLHA during treatment, MMM, and HBC visits. Medical treatment would be conducted at the referral hospital rather than by the home visit teams, consistent with the increased emphasis on the referral hospital as the center for care.

The more local organization of these small home-visit teams means that transport costs should be greatly reduced. The challenge will be to maintain close linkages between the teams and the health providers at the referral hospital. Any adoption of this plan will need careful monitoring to ensure that the organizational challenges can be met.

The reliance on NGOs to provide HBC leaves gaps in some ODs. Filling these gaps will not be simple. Khmer HIV/AIDS NGO Alliance (KHANA) acts as an umbrella organization for these NGOs. Although it does not have official activities aimed at forming new NGOs, it has helped some PLHA to become a community-based organization and finally an NGO. It is not easy, however, to communicate what it means to be an NGO, and the responsibilities that go with that role.

Outreach or transport?

With funds for HBC being limited, organizations must choose how much they spend on salaries for outreach staff (including per diems for volunteers) and how much they spend on subsidizing PLHA transport to the referral hospital. PLHA who are on ART must, in most locations, go to the referral hospital every month for a check-up and a new supply of ART drugs. (An exception is those getting treatment from MSF, who after 6 months start getting a 2 month supply of antiretroviral drugs.) These travel costs are lessening somewhat as more sites provide OI/ART. PLHA are being referred back to the treatment center nearest their home, and so do not have to travel as far. But travel costs for clinical visits are still a major expense for many PLHA.

For now, some HBC services overwhelmingly put the emphasis on funding their outreach teams (e.g., the ratio of spending on outreach vs. PLHA transport in one case was 36:1). This may be the correct priority, but organizations should at least be conscious that they are making this choice. Reducing the size of HBC teams, as discussed above, may help direct more money towards PLHA transport.

IV.3. PLHA involvement

The long-term nature of AIDS treatment makes it essential that PLHA get involved in their own treatment, the dissemination of educational messages, peer support, and in guiding hospital activities. Increased involvement can change "the role of PLHA from being passive consumers of health care to becoming partners in care provision" and "build their confidence and pride."[14]

IV. Linkages to the Community

For the running of the CoC, in general 2 PLHA volunteers help with the convening of the MMM and as drug educators and counselors in the OI/ART clinic. These 2 volunteers are also members of the CoC-CC, and bring messages from the MMM to the attention of this group. This feedback is critical for the proper functioning of the CoC. If funding is available, PLHA may also help as counselors in the VCCT service, as guides in the hospital, and in taking patient histories in pre-consultation interviews.

CPN+ and Self-help groups

Capacity building and advocacy for PLHA is promoted by CPN+. An educated group of PLHA have improved HIV/AIDS care in many countries, and continued education will help Cambodian PLHA to be informed about a wide range of issues, including those associated with moving into 2nd line ART regimens. CPN+ staff therefore train PLHA in education and advocacy skills, and organize activities to increase PLHA visibility during special events. They meet nationally with government and NGO staff, via representation on all major coordination bodies, and at the local level with self-help group leaders. All provincial CPN+ staff are themselves PLHA.

Self-help groups can help PLHA to solve their own problems and provide each other with support. CPN+ and other local NGOs (often those providing HBC) help PLHA to form self-help groups. These groups can help PLHA to solve their own problems and provide each other with support. In general, funding for these groups is poor, and thus their activities are limited in areas such as income-generating activities or provision of food.

With little or no money the self-help groups can, however, help compensate for any limitations in MMM capacity. Representatives from self-help groups often bring concerns to the MMM. The groups also pass information to HBC teams to help them in identifying hidden PLHA cases.

How NCHADS coordinates with local partners

In encouraging the involvement of PLHA and NGOs, NCHADS balances the desires for coherent organization on the one hand and local ownership on the other. Inevitably, using local partners results in variability, depending on the availability and quality of NGOs in different ODs. Central coordination of NGO efforts helps minimize this variation, and thus ensures that community and PLHA involvement — two central elements of the CoC — are implemented fully.

NCHADS immediately realized that NGOs would have to pick up much of the burden in terms of community and PLHA involvement,[15] while it kept the funding of medical treatment as its first priority. If NCHADS did not take this approach, and tried to take on all of these tasks, there would be a great risk of drawing human resources away from other medical activities, and thus weakening other parts of the health system.

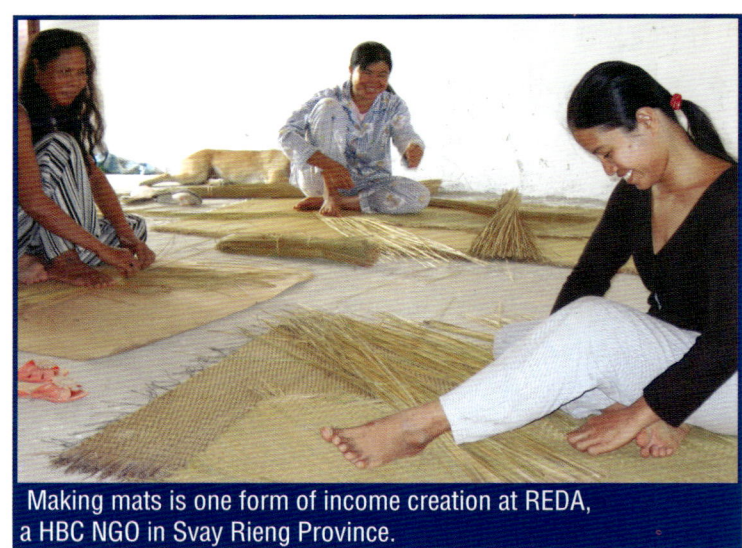

Making mats is one form of income creation at REDA, a HBC NGO in Svay Rieng Province.

V. The Challenges and Potential of Expansion

V.1. Resource constraints: what gives when there is less money?

Country-wide expansion of the CoC means that many ODs must adopt the CoC and especially HBC activities with little or no support from large NGOs. It is important to know whether this is a viable strategy, as full coverage by the CoC relies upon it.

The one indisputable difference between ODs supported by large NGOs and those without such support is money: the unsupported ODs have less of it. The consequences of this for the CoC are more difficult to tease apart.

NCHADS funds the core services of the CoC — most notably the training and incentives necessary for essential medical care. NGOs often finance extra activities that help support these core services. This was particularly important in the initial OD of Moung Russey for two reasons: it helped establish an initial, high standard; and it provided the extra resources so that this first OD could absorb the subsequent training needs of the other ODs.

Setting an initial example is very important. ODs with less support have many CoC staff members who will be overworked: their work on the CoC exceeds what might be expected based on their compensation alone. These staff have adopted a service-delivery model that is country-devised and country-owned, and has already shown great success in other provinces. They are determined to reproduce that success in their own location.

NCHADS now faces the challenge of sustaining this motivation. Over time, activities seen as optional, such as volunteers to show PLHA around the hospital, or extra funding for general laboratory activities, may be acknowledged as essential for long-term sustainability of the increased effort. Additional funds will also be needed, especially for community support activities and to sustain capacity building by using refresher trainings, exchanges and study tours, and supervision.

ODs with little support will also have to work hard to build sufficient links to the community. **Several healthcare administrators cited the most difficult aspect of establishing a CoC as not the technical challenges but ensuring community participation.** NCHADS welcomes NGOs based on their expertise in reaching communities, and this is where several NGOs have put their greatest efforts.

NGOs can support HBC teams and social workers who cover areas without HBC. Within the referral hospital, NGOs can increase the number of PLHA involved, including PLHA guides, increase OI/ART team size, and provide funds so that not just one but all of the staff in a given unit (e.g., TB) can be trained. Finally, NGO staff can act as ongoing monitors. Without their participation, it is even more important to have ongoing monitoring and evaluation.

Of the ODs examined here, Neak Loeung has the least resources and support. The main, consistent concern in this OD was the relative lack of funding for PLHA activities. More money was needed to pay for PLHA transportation costs (to appointments and MMM), for food at MMM, and for enough HBC teams. As discussed above, NCHADS considers it the role of civil society to supply many of these functions. However, it was clear that the main components of the CoC had been successfully established. **This suggests that moving ahead with the CoC, even when not everything appears to be ready, is a risk worth taking when there is overall clarity of purpose.**

V.2. Spillovers: Can the CoC cause general health system strengthening?

Worldwide, there has been a huge influx of financial resources into HIV/AIDS treatment activities, but has this benefited other parts of the health systems? The Global Fund for AIDS, TB and Malaria (GFATM) has recognized that general health system capacity is essential for providing OI/ART, resulting in the 5th Round funding cycle being earmarked for system strengthening. GFATM is also sponsoring an evaluation of whether its own disbursements are leading to system strengthening in Benin, Ethiopia, and Mali.[16] Evidence in those

V. The Challenges and Potential of Expansion

countries thus far is similar to the findings reported here from Cambodia: that the limited time since implementation means that such spillovers are currently more a matter of promising potential.

CoC activities could in theory improve the rest of the healthcare system in a number of ways. These include:

- ♦ improved management techniques that are devised as part of the CoC, and picked up by other parts of the healthcare system;
- ♦ increased technical ability of OI/ART clinicians that these clinicians use, or train their colleagues to use, when treating non-PLHA;
- ♦ increased utilization of other hospital services when PLHA tell their community that the referral hospital provides good care;
- ♦ improved general laboratory and pharmacy operations, if common equipment and supplies are purchased using HIV resources, and if training in HIV laboratory operations and HIV pharmacy supply management is used to improve the general services;
- ♦ improved work ethic of OI/ART team that spreads to other hospital workers.

In general there was some evidence for all of these spillovers. At the very least, the CoC brings more PLHA into the hospitals. For example, in Moung Russey the CoC consultations now represent up to 25% of all monthly consultations. This breaks the cycle in which patients do not come to hospitals because of a perception of poor clinical practice, and doctors cannot improve their clinical practice because too few patients come to see them. In Neak Loeung, the enthusiasm and hard work of CoC staff (even before salary supplements started) has reportedly acted as a model for other services.

Not surprisingly, evidence for spillovers was most obvious in Moung Russey, where the CoC has been established the longest and where FHI subsidized additional trainings, equipment, and renovations that built general system capacity as much as HIV-specific care. The next greatest impact of HIV-related equipment and supply purchases has come in hospitals that were initially the most deficient in basic supplies (e.g., without adequate fridges, mixers, furniture, and a spectrophotometer). HIV/AIDS is also forcing hospitals to confront the need to track patients over time. Although this issue was not examined in depth, it is expected that the CoC is helping the Cambodian healthcare system to meet the challenges of chronic care.

A rise in the number of non-PLHA patients was not evident to most hospital workers. This may reflect the relatively short time since CoC implementation began. For this spillover to occur, a series of steps are required. Training must first take hold in the OI/ART team, then be transferred to other healthcare workers, change the perception about quality of care that filters out to the community, and finally induce behavior change in the community. Each step takes time.

Healthcare workers also said that some issues of general health system capacity (such as the lack of an adequate ambulance service) remained as leading barriers to good care for PLHA. The extent of spillovers was thought to be generally limited because even the CoC, as a disease-specific service-delivery model, is perceived as somewhat vertical.

This perception may change over time if international partners embrace a more inclusive vision of HIV/AIDS care. After all, PLHA often use general facilities (general lab, general medications, etc) whereas non-PLHA rarely use specialized HIV-funded equipment. Physical infrastructure also takes time to adapt to a more integrated approach: in many referral hospitals the laboratories were previously divided into separate facilities for each different major disease.

The division between general and HIV facilities still exists for laboratory and pharmacy services in many referral hospitals. And drug supplies are often paid for by two different pots of money (HIV and general Ministry of Health) and maintained by two different staff members working independently. In Moung Russey, a single person purchases HIV drugs from NCHADS and other drugs from the Central Medical Store (CMS), and the HIV testing and general lab tests are in one location. Hopefully other ODs will follow this more integrated model as their CoC adoption progresses.

Inducing an increase in spillovers will take a movement in both resources and ways of thinking. Vertical organization has been the predominant practice for many years. Thus the concept of spillovers — that one sector might benefit other sectors in the hospital — was not widespread. Financial resources would certainly help change this. If HIV donors funded services that PLHA share with others, such as general laboratory equipment and reagents, then this would provide a firm push towards integration.

VI. The Future of the CoC

VI.1. Areas for future expansion

The CoC continues to adapt to changing circumstances, even as it retains a core of consistent services. Below are listed some of the areas that are adding further value to the existing CoC integrated services.

OI/ART—former district hospitals and second-line treatments

CoC treatment occurs at the referral hospital. Although health center staff take part in HBC teams, they have limited knowledge about HIV/AIDS care and treatment. In the future, however, it may be possible to transfer CoC skills and HIV/AIDS treatment to some former district hospitals. The teaching involved in this transfer would present a valuable opportunity to link former district hospitals with their referral hospital.

For ART, second - and third-line regimens are needed when first-line options fail. But these alternative regimens are expensive and generally far more complex for patients to take.[17] By September 2005, 1.9% of those on ART in Cambodia were taking a regimen that included a protease inhibitor. The size of this group is expected to grow.

Social sectors and the CoC

Current plans with the National Aids Authority (NAA) call for increased communication and planning with other sectors – especially education, social welfare, and religion – so that they can add additional elements to the CoC. Impact mitigation will occur in collaboration with the Ministry of Social Welfare, Youth, and Rehabilitation (MoSWYR). Greater support (food and school supplies) for orphans and vulnerable children (OVC) will probably be the first step.

Secondary prevention

PLHA who are on ART, or their partners, may think that the PLHA are now cured. This has prompted NCHADS and KHANA to combine care and prevention efforts. Condom distribution to PLHA, and education of HIV-discordant couples, will increase with the expansion of the CoC. These issues are an important part of the MMM agenda.

TB/HIV

Approximately 10% of TB patients in Cambodia are HIV positive, and up to 40% of PLHA enrolled for OI/ART have active TB infections. The CoC provides one way to link TB and HIV treatment activities, which are run by separate government agencies.[18]

TB/HIV joint activities are already part of the CoC. Uptake of HIV testing by TB patients is, however, low, as many TB patients get their treatment at health centers where VCCT is not available.

CENAT and NCHADS have agreed on several common strategies (including transport incentives, transport of blood samples, and mobile VCCT staff in specific geographic areas) to increase HIV testing of this population. HBC teams also have the potential to bridge any gap between the treatment activities in the communities. Finally, treatment guidelines for TB/HIV will no doubt continue to evolve in line with international standards, so that under certain conditions concurrent treatment may be used.

PMTCT

Expanding PMTCT to all CoC sites is a very high priority. Detecting mothers' infections during ANC is important not only for preventing

VI. The Future of the CoC

infection of the unborn child, but also for getting the mother into treatment when her disease is less advanced. This way, she will have a much greater opportunity to benefit from medical attention. Although the initial focus is on the mother, under the family care approach the full range of CoC services are made available to all family members.

Just less than half of all pregnant women in Cambodia come to at least one ANC visit. Of these, 52% have an HIV test during their first ANC visit. There are several ways that this number may be boosted in the future. Besides expanding to more ODs, PMTCT services may devise ways to prioritize the testing of those who live further away and must leave early, and perhaps even consider opt-out HIV testing. NCMCH and NCHADS have a coordinated plan for PMTCT so that there is a single, coherent message encouraging mothers to get tested.

VI.2. Financial resources, local leadership, and will

The CoC demonstrates that Cambodia has implementing capacity if there are financial resources, leadership, and will. The staff who made the CoC happen were previously underutilized: they ran important prevention campaigns but have now added a complex set of treatment activities to their portfolio with relatively little expansion in their numbers. This is the broadest level lesson that arises from the CoC. Where there are financial resources, leadership, and political will, human capacity emerges and flourishes.

Appendix A: Interview subjects

H.E Dr Mam Bun Heng, Secretary of State for Health, Ministry of Health

H.E Dr Mean Chhi Vun, Director, NCHADS

Dr Michael O'Leary, Country Representative, WHO Cambodia

Dr Massimo Ghidinelli, HIV/AIDS Technical Adviser, WHO Cambodia

Dr Nicole Seguy, HIV/AIDS Medical Officer, WHO Cambodia

Mr Lyma Virakrith, Deputy Director of RH and OI/ART team leader, Neak Loeung

MA Neang Samith, Chief of VCCT, counselor, Neak Loeung

Dr Long Nhoeuth, OD Director, Neak Loeung

MA Ouk Sundeth, CoC coordinator, Neak Loeung

Mr Ouk Siphon, HBC team member at Preak Hasay "B" health center

Dr Ly Hour Sour, Chief of medicine ward and communicable diseases, OI/ART clinician, Neak Loeung

Mr Ouk Oeurn, Deputy Director of PHD, and chair of provincial AIDS secretariat in Prey Veng Province

MA Deap Veasna, PAO Manager, PHD Prey Veng,

Dr Ung Soeung Kang, PAO Manager, PHD Svay Rieng

Dr Orng Sophat, Deputy Director of PHD Svay Rieng

Mr Nop Nara, CoC coordinator, Svay Rieng PHD

Mr Chea Sarith, President of WOMEN (Women Organization for Modern Economy and Nursing)

Ms Long Socheat, HBC volunteer with WOMEN, Ba Phnom, Prey Veng

Mr Prom Chan, HBC volunteer with WOMEN, Ba Phnom, Prey Veng

Dr Chea Sorphoan, OD CoC Coordinator and OD Technical Bureau Officer, Svay Rieng

Dr Chan Dara, Acting RH director, Svay Rieng

Dr La Kim Khemarin, Chief of general medical services and OI/ART for adults, Svay Rieng RH

MA An Sophy, Pediatric OI/ART, Svay Rieng RH

MA So Boran, Deputy of OPD, chief of Psychiatry ward, Svay Rieng RH

Ms Sok Thary, VCCT lab technician, Svay Rieng RH

Mr Sok Savuth, Chief of VCCT and Counselor, Svay Rieng RH

Ms Ea Channimol, Chief of General Laboratory, Deputy of Pharmacy, Svay Rieng RH

Ms Keo Sarady, Assistant with CPN+ in Svay Rieng

Mr Poa Sovanna, Assistant to Executive Director,
Rural Economic Development Association (REDA), Svay Rieng

Mr Pok Thoeun, Program Manager, REDA, Svay Rieng

Dr Samreth Sovannarith, Head of HBC Sub-unit at NCHADS

Dr Masaya Kato, HIV/AIDS technical adviser, CARE Cambodia

Ms Touch Savun, VCCT at Moundoul Mouie HC and PAO staff, Siem Reap RH

Ms Thong Ramy, PMTCT coordinator, MCH staff, Siem Reap RH

Mr Chhay Tich, RH director, CoC committee member, OI/ART team leader of ESTHER, Siem Reap RH

Dr Chy Say, OI/ART physician, Assistant Project Coordinator, MSF, Siem Reap

MA Tan Ruon, TB ward physician, Siem Reap RH

Mr Un Phay, Nurse and registration in OI/ART team, Siem Reap RH

Ms Tan Kim Siv, Pharmacist, Chief of Drug Bureau for PHD, and for ESTHER HIV drugs, Siem Reap RH

Mr Kim Sour, Programme Officer, Salvation Center Cambodia (SCC, a HBC NGO), Siem Reap

Mr San Pun, Monk team leader, SCC, Siem Reap

Mr Im Oeun, Monk team leader, SCC, Siem Reap

Mr Hot Kim Heat, Field worker, SCC, Siem Reap

Ms Chhun Chhairorn, CPN+ Coordinator, Siem Reap

Mr Meng Mresna, CPN+ Assistant, Siem Reap

Mr Kazumi Akao, Technical Adviser, HIV/AIDS Home Care program, Angkor Hospital for Children, Siem Reap

Dr Soeung Seitaboth, Pediatrician and HIV/AIDS consultant, Angkor Hospital for Children, Siem Reap

Dr Kuy Sok, Deputy Director of Battambang PHD and PHD CoC Technical Support Team leader, Battambang PHD

Mr Ret Rithy, GIPA field worker, Battambang

MA Huy Nory, MCH physician, Moung Russey RH

Dr Ho Sidara, Chief maternity ward, chief of PMTCT, Moung Russey RH

Mr Menh Vongchan, VCCT controller, Moung Russey RH

Mrs Eap Mealea, Lab Primary, Moung Russey RH

Dr Peov Sovannarin, OD Coordinator, OI/ART team leader, Moung Russey RH

Dr So Sok, RH Director, Deputy director of CoC-CC, RH CoC Coordinator, Moung Russey RH

Mr Sorth Vathana, Chief of Health Center in grounds of Moung Russey RH

Mr Nheub Bunthoeurn, Program Manager, Kien Kes Health Education Network HBC NGO, Battambang

Mr Matthew Warner-Smith, UNAIDS Cambodia

Dr Chawalit Natpratan, Country Director, FHI Cambodia

Mrs Tess Prombuth, Director, Care and Treatment, FHI Cambodia

Mr Heng Sokrithy, Country Coordinator, CPN+

Dr Chhim Sarath, Senior Program Officer, KHANA

Dr Chin Sedtha, Assistant Project Officer, HIV/AIDS, UNICEF

References

[1] NCHADS. 2003. *Continuum of Care for People Living with HIV/AIDS. Operational Framework. 1st Edition.*

[2] Dhaliwal, M., and T. Ellman for the International HIV/AIDS Alliance. 2003. *Improving Access to Anti-retroviral Treatment in Cambodia.*

[3] Attawell, K., and J. Mundy for WHO and DFID. 2003. *Provision of Antiretroviral Therapy in Resource-Limited Settings: A Review of Experience Up to August 2003.*

[4] Oliveira-Cruz, V., et al. 2004. *The Brazilian HIV/AIDS 'Success Story' – Can Others Do It? Trop. Med. Intnl. Health. vol. 9:292–297.*

[5] NCHADS, WHO and FHI. 2004. *Cambodia Cares: Implementing a Continuum of Care for PLHA, including ART, in Moung Russey, Cambodia.*

[6] Brink, A.-K., NCHADS, and FHI. 2005. *Continuum of Care for Rapid Scale-Up of Care and Treatment Services for People Living with HIV/AIDS. Proceedings of an Inter-Country Field-Oriented Workshop, Battambang Province, Kingdom of Cambodia.*

[7] Schneider, H., et al. 2004. *Health System Strengthening and ART Scaling Up: Challenges and Opportunities.*

[8] WHO Department of HIV/AIDS. 2003. *A Public Health Approach for Scaling Up Antiretroviral (ARV) Treatment: A Toolkit for Programme Managers.*

[9] International HIV/AIDS Alliance. 2002. *Improving Access to HIV/AIDS-Related Treatment.*

[10] Kober, K., and W. van Damme. 2003. *The Early Steps of the Global Fund in Cambodia.*

[11] Wilkinson, D., and the International HIV/AIDS Alliance. *2000. An Evaluation of the MoH/NGO Home Care Programme for People with HIV/AIDS in Cambodia.*

[12] Fletcher, G. 2003. *Voluntary Confidential Counseling and Testing in Cambodia: An Overview.*

[13] Mukherjee, J., et al. *Access to Antiretroviral Treatment and Care: The Experience of the HIV Equity Initiative, Cange, Haiti. A Case Study in the WHO series Perspectives and Practice in Antiretroviral Treatment.*

[14] Kumphitak, A., et al. *Involvement of People Living with HIV/AIDS in Treatment Preparedness in Thailand. A Case Study in the WHO series Perspectives and Practice in Antiretroviral Treatment.*

[15] Wilkinson, D. 2005. *A Healthy Partnership – a Case Study of the MoH Contract to KHANA for Disbursement of World Bank Funds for HIV/AIDS in Cambodia.*

[16] Stillman, K. and S. Bennett. 2005. *Systemwide Effects of the Global Fund: Interim Findings from Three Country Studies.*

[17] MSF. 2004. *Rapid Expansion; Emerging Challenges. Briefing Document.*

[18] Wilkinson, D. 2001. *Linking HIV and TB – Underlying Issues to Consider When Scaling Integration of HIV and TB Services in Cambodia.*

Notes